# Traditional Hair Care and Scalp Care Methods

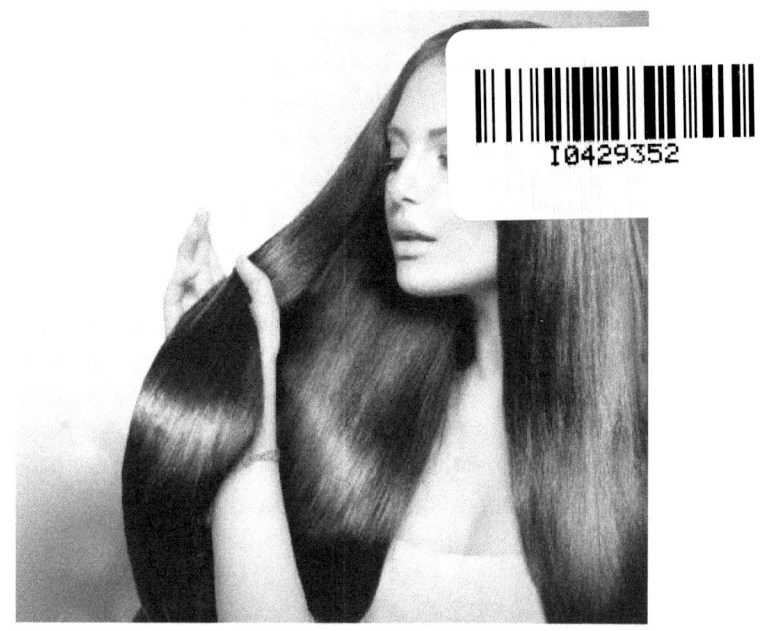

## Natural Ancient Ways to Keep Your Hair and Scalp Healthy

### Dueep Jyot Singh

### Mendon Cottage Books

### Health Learning Series

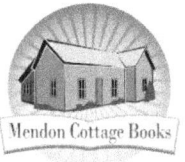

*JD-Biz Publishing*

**Download Free Books!**

http://MendonCottageBooks.com

## All Rights Reserved.

No part of this publication may be reproduced in any form or by any means, including scanning, photocopying, or otherwise without prior written permission from JD-Biz Corp Copyright © 2016

All Images Licensed by Fotolia and 123RF.

**Disclaimer**

The information is this book is provided for informational purposes only. The information is believed to be accurate as presented based on research by the author.

The author or publisher is not responsible for the use or safety of any procedure or treatment mentioned in this book. The author or publisher is not responsible for errors or omissions that may exist.

### Our books are available at

1. Amazon.com
2. Barnes and Noble
3. Itunes
4. Kobo
5. Smashwords
6. Google Play Books

## Download Free Books!

## http://MendonCottageBooks.com

# Table of Contents

Introduction ................................................................. 5

Herbal Nourishing Remedies .................................... 10

    Traditional Gooseberry Jam .................................. 11

    Traditional Way to Make Gooseberry Mirabba .................. 13

    How to Eat This Jam .......................................... 13

Hair Fall .................................................... 16

    Gooseberry Water .......................................... 20

    Gooseberry Oil – Natural Conditioner ....................... 21

    First Preparation Method – Traditional ...................... 21

    The Second Method ........................................ 22

Curing Dandruff ............................................ 25

    Lemons .................................................... 26

    Treating Lice ............................................... 28

    Traditional Soap Nut Shampoo .............................. 28

    Yogurt Shampoo – Natural Hair Darkener .................... 32

    Pepper and Salt Hair ........................................ 33

    Lemon Oil Supporting Treatment ........................... 34

    Final Rinse ................................................ 36

    Fullers Earth Shampoo ...................................... 37

Chickpea – Gram Flour Shampoo ............................................. 38

Baldness ................................................................................... 39

Traditional Natural Hair Dye .................................................. 40

Henna Dye ................................................................................ 41

Conclusion ................................................................................ 43
Author Bio ................................................................................ 45
Publisher ................................................................................... 56

# Introduction

Since ancient times, the sign of a genuine natural beauty was one who had long, silky, healthy, and shiny hair. No wonder they were called the crowning glory atop the head of a beautiful woman. Men also were very particular about haircare in ancient times, when in Phoenicia and ancient Greece, Babylon, and Egypt, they put a sweet smelling cone on their heads, and wrapped their hair around it in traditional hairstyles.

This book is going to tell you all about the natural methods in which you can take care of your hair. Apart from this, it is going to tell you all about the prevention and cure of a number of problems related to the head, scalp, and hair and how they have been cured traditionally.

Along with this, you are going to get plenty of information on how you can take care of your hair through a proper and healthy diet. Traditional antiaging remedies and recipes are going to be given to you, taken from all over the world and all of them time-tested and ancient.

It does not matter where you are; haircare is something which has to be a part of your daily routine. Once upon a time, fashion conscious people did not bother much about shampooing or cleaning their hair. Instead, they got their slaves and their servants to brush out their hair, 100 times everyday nodded to get rid of all the dirt and grime, and because everybody had equally grimy hair in their vicinity, nobody bothered much about the smell of highly perfumed unguents applied on the hair.

In ancient Egypt men and women of high rank, shaved their heads and wore wigs instead. Good way to keep their scalps problem free, but they would suffer from skin problems because of those tightfitting wigs and the fungi breeding under them in a muggy atmosphere.

Scalp problems include dandruff, itching, skin ailments, and even lice. Lice unfortunately have been with us since day one itself, and the problem of cooties attacking the scalp of school going children has been one, which every responsible parent has to face sometime or the other.

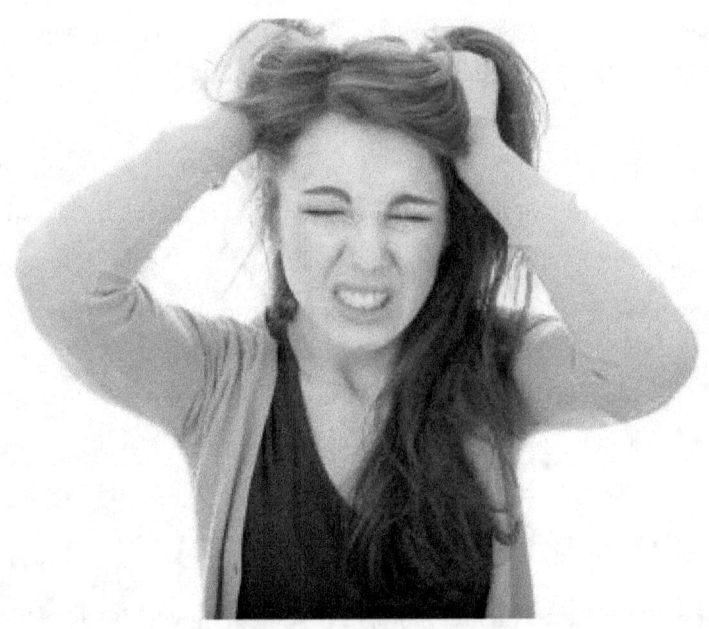

And to make sure that I do not have an itching scalp, full of dandruff, I applied some warm oil, and massaged it into my skull, scalp, and hair, right before I switched on the computer and started on this book. By the time I finish it, all that oil will have been absorbed by the scalp, and all the grime collected in the oil.

After that, I am going to wash my hair with natural shampoos, which I am going to tell you. Also, you are going to get to know about natural hair conditioners, and other factors which are essential to keep your hair healthy, beautiful, silky, smooth, and so soft to touch, and good to feel.

In between this duration, I am going to get up and stretch my legs perhaps 3 hours from now. And then I am going to plaster a paste of dried gooseberry powder made in water all over the scalp. When it has dried, that means I have made sure that I am not going to suffer from any graying of my hair ever, even though I will never see 45 again.

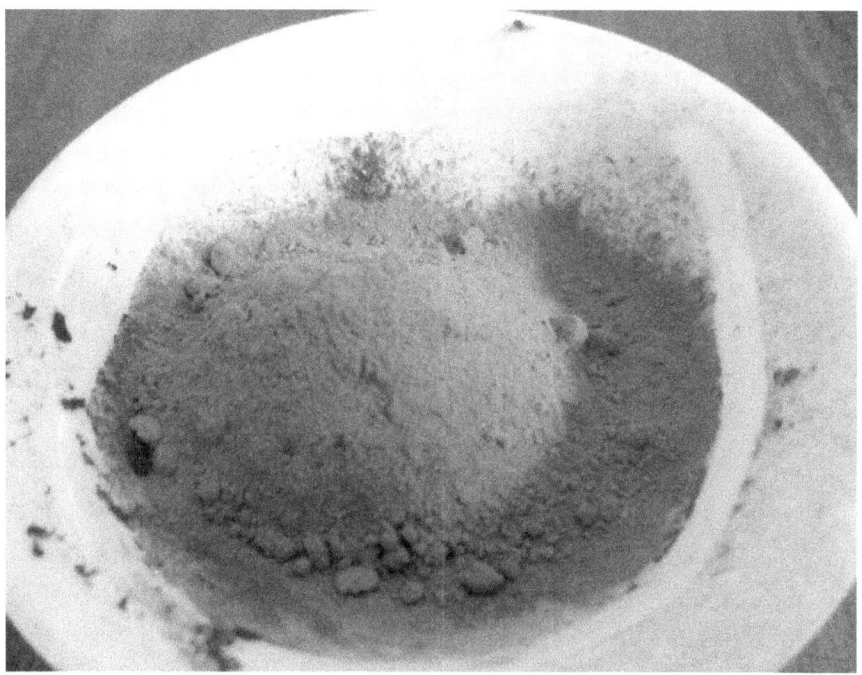

**Natural gooseberry powder - Never mix traditional herbs or natural products in plastic, synthetic, or even Melamine bowls, always use glass or porcelain, as far as possible.**

This is the gooseberry which I apply on my hair, and so I am not bother much about how pure it is. That is because I am using it externally and not internally. But real powdered gooseberry is going to be edible, – made out of powder dry fruits – and I am going to take a teaspoonful of it, every night before going to sleep, stirred in a glass full of warm water, to get rid of the toxins, and to stop the graying process right now.

That means if I managed to live up to my seventies and eighties, at least. I will not be as gray as Brother Gray Wolf.

I greeted my younger brother on his birthday a couple of days ago by telling him that he looked like my Elder brother what with his hair growing gray on his temples and his once sleek black head now looking like the fur of an old mouse.

And to top it off, there I was, 3 years older with just the barest modicum or not very visible gray in my head. And he knows very well that I do not dye my hair. He had a happy fuming and fulminating birthday.

This was of course, in keeping with the traditional sibling psychology of show your affection to your siblings by twisting their tails whenever you can, and being as rude as possible. That reassured him that I was in top form and he had not to worry about my health, mental, emotional, or physical!

In fact he does look like my older brother. But then he started growing distinguished and gray in his thirties. It is a matter of great chagrin to women that men can go gray, and still look distinguished, but women do not seem to look so good, with wrinkles and gray hair.

I admit to having a couple of white hairs, but they sprang up, because I had gone out in the winter sun without covering my head for a couple of hours yesterday. So they had to bleach. I have left them strictly alone, because if I pull them out, the follicles around them are going to go gray.

Instead, get your hair follicles back to normal with natural traditional methods which are going to keep your system healthy as well as your hair.

# Herbal Nourishing Remedies

I am now introducing a fruit, which is not only going to solve your graying problems, but is going to keep you healthy.

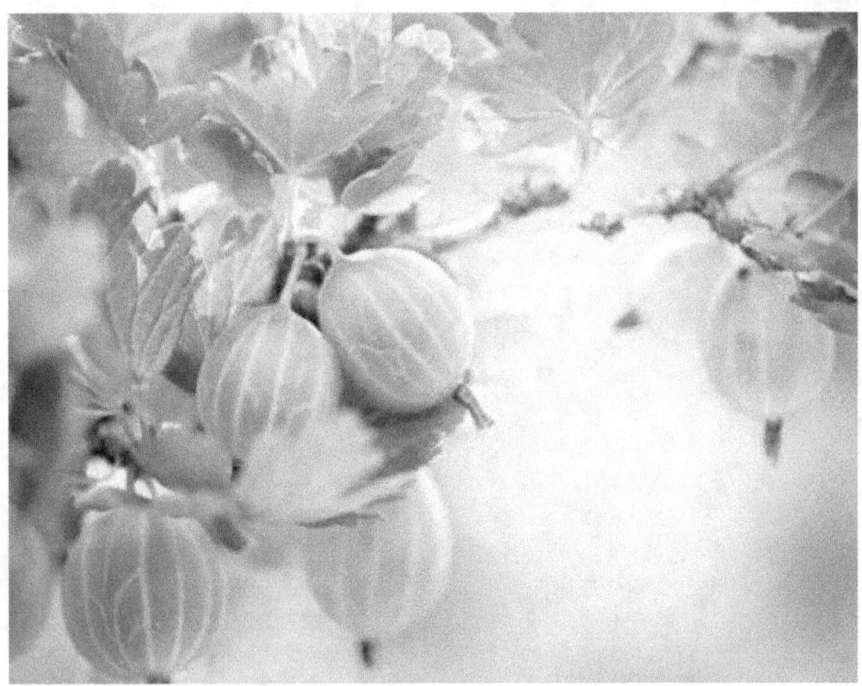

**Gooseberries**

The herbs and fruit given here in these remedies are available all over the world. One of them is one of nature's most powerful antioxidant, antibacterial, antispasmodic, rich source of vitamin C, fiber, calcium, phosphorus, iron, carotene, and amino acids like riboflavin.

It is called a gooseberry. – Emblica officianalis. The next few pages are going to tell you all about traditional recipes, made for good health, as well as for haircare, with the use of this particular herb/fruit.

You can either eat it raw or in dried form. It has a rather sour taste. It is an excellent source of vitamin C, and that is why we spent all our childhood, gnawing on these raw fruit purloined from the neighbors' gardens, even if our own gooseberry fruit laden trees were groaning under the burden of gooseberries. But then we knew that some of our friends would be stalking our fruit, so that was all right.

# Traditional Gooseberry Jam

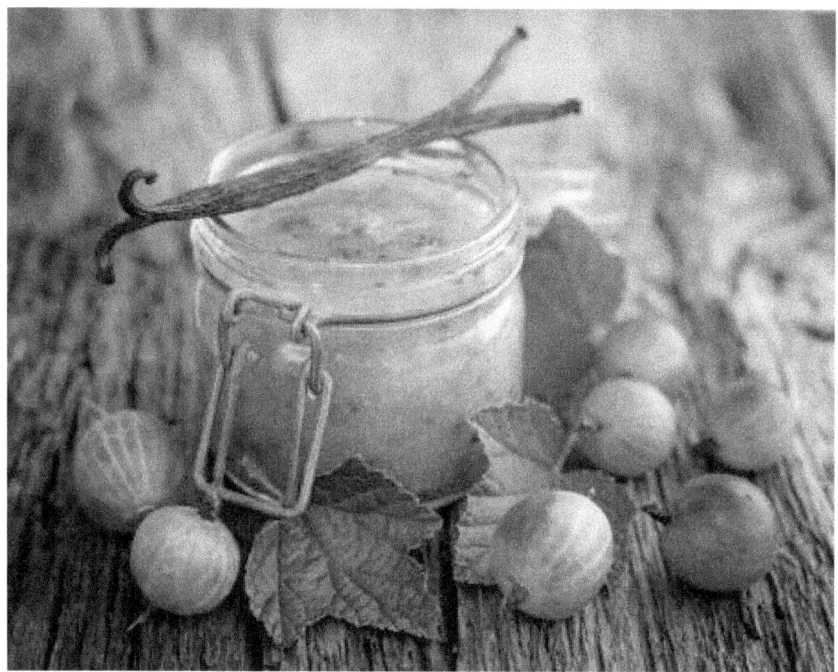

**Traditional gooseberry jam is always made in honey, and stored in a glass bottle.**

According to the ancients, gooseberry was excellent for the brain, eyes, blood circulation, temperature regulation, heart, liver, digestion, and other parts of the body.

This jam was traditionally made in South and Central Asia, and the Caucasian region like Georgia and Azerbaijan with spices, honey, sugar, and fruit. It was, and is still called *Mirabba* traditionally or Varenye in Russia.

Traditional gooseberry jam was made by every self-respecting grandmother throughout the year, down the ages whenever the gooseberries were in season or they were just powdered, so that they could be used out of season.

Naturally, gooseberry powder is an excellent antioxidant and amazing Anti aging rejuvenating natural material. Also, expectant mothers were given this fruit so that they could enjoy plenty of good health, and have healthy children with a really strong immune system.

You can also have it in pickled form. Do not take it in large quantities in a day like say more than 3 gooseberries. Even though we had anywhere between 3 to 4 every day when we were kids. But then our digestive system was used to digesting sticks and stones like ostriches and goats.

One gooseberry fruit from this jam was enough for adults and half for children given in the morning every day on an empty stomach, and then nothing given to them for an hour afterwards. After that, you could have your breakfast. This was the best brain growth food for children, and good nervous system growth material for adults.

This was normally fed to every member of the family in the summer. In ancient times, it was covered with a thin layer of silver foil so that you did not have to worry about any similar material and mineral deficiency either!

Also, it would cool your system, in the summer, so that you did not suffer from summer related problems, dizziness, fatigue, and lethargy.

This was given to a number of patients suffering from diabetes because it had pure honey in it.

## Traditional Way to Make Gooseberry Mirabba

Take 500 g of green clean gooseberries. Grade them or you can leave them whole, as you wish. Now put them into a glass jar. Do not use plastic jars or any other 21st-century container. Now put just enough honey on this pulp to soak it all up. After this, you are going to put this in the sun for 4 to 5 hours, every day for the next 10 days.

In this manner, you are going to get a natural traditional jam, with all the goodness of honey incorporated in it, after being cooked in the sun.

Allow 2 more days and it is ready to eat. This is the best traditional recipe, because nowadays, these gooseberries are cooked in sugar syrup on fire and that is a pity. The ancients had a great trust in the power of the sun and its healing rays in order to cook food and to get all the natural goodness of all the elements in this process.

## How to Eat This Jam

If you have grated it, you are going to take two teaspoons full, first thing in the morning on an empty stomach. If you have preserved the full fruit, you are going to take one, if you are an adult, and half if you are a child. Do not eat anything one hour after eating this so that you have plenty of chance for it to do its best work and get assimilated into your system early in the morning. Eat this for the next month, especially in the summer.

You can also drink one glass of warm milk, 15 minutes after you have taken this dose for breakfast. This is going to give you the best effects when taken in March, April, and September, October.

If you happen to be a student or happen to be using your brainpower more than you use your muscle power, this is going to be particularly beneficial to you, because this is considered to be the best and oldest brain health-food, especially when it is combined with honey and cooked in the sun.

Also, if you find yourself suffering from stress and tension, you may find yourself calming down. It is rich in vitamin C, A, calcium, and Iron.

This is the only fruit in the world, which still retains its minerals and vitamins even after it has been cooked or dried.

If you really do not have the time to prepare it, this natural way, but have access to fresh gooseberries, you can grate it and take 2 teaspoons with one teaspoonful of honey. This is excellent for getting rid of chronic ailments of the stomach.

Now we come to powdered gooseberry. This is where we come to haircare, especially if you are wondering about the health of your hair, unnatural, graying, and hair fall.

Take one teaspoonful of powdered gooseberry in two mouthfuls of water just before you go to sleep. This is going to stop the graying process completely. Also, you are going to find your skin glowing, because of the vitamin C. Incidentally, if you are suffering from a harsh voice,[1] it is going to soften your tone and make it melodious again.

---

[1] Talking about croaks – I remember picking up a ridiculous escapist novel because I did not have anything better to do, and the heroine had a "lovely croak", with a voice like a cat yowling at the moon. She repeated it so many times in the book, that when the heroine spoke in her lovely croak – yes, those words 8 times in the next 15 days, that book hit a wall to be put in the dustbin the next morning – And the author tried to persuade us that the hero thought it attractive. I guess, this is on par with the absurd videos on YouTube teaching you how to have a harsh supposedly attractive voice, as if you are suffering from a cold. But do not worry, this idiocy is not restricted to the 21st-century, Barbara Cartland's mother Polly was born with a melodious voice, but as a child, she caught a cold and was told not to speak and rest her throat and tongue. In keeping with the intellectual power of girls of those days – compulsive motor mouths –, she talked and yelled and chattered and for the rest of her life, she had a harsh , shrill nasal voice, which sounded as if she had a cold.

# Hair Fall

So many of us are so obsessed with hair fall, that we find ourselves stressing out the moment we find our brush full of hair. This young girl is going to get into a tizzy right now. What she does not know is that this much hair fall is natural and expected because hair also have a limited age upon the scalp and when it is time for them to fall, they are going to drop out of the follicles.

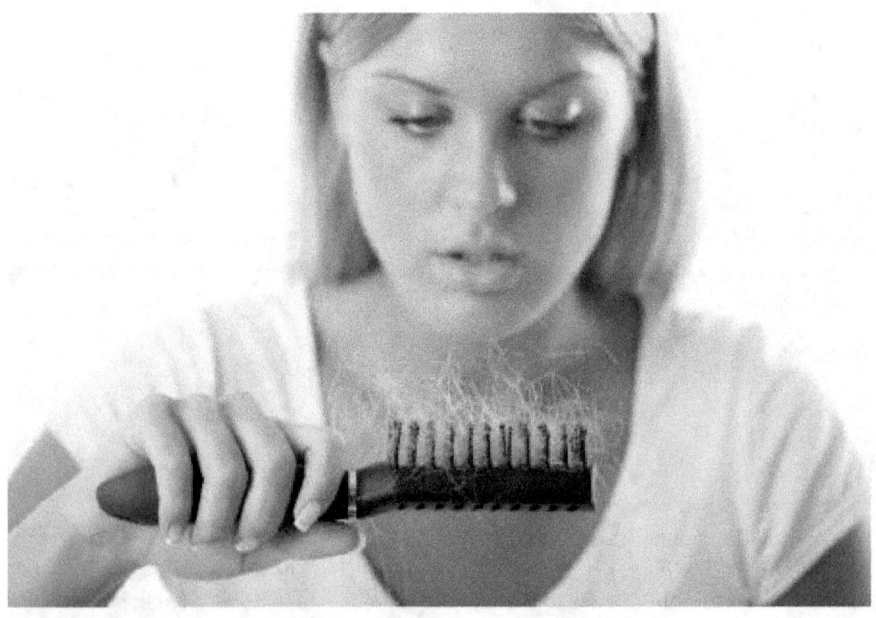

It is only when you find your hair coming out in large amounts, especially in chunks, that it is time to begin worrying, because apart from stress, this can be a warning signal given by your body that there is something wrong in your system somewhere, and either there is a mineral or nutritional deficiency or it may be symptomatic of some other potentially serious problem.

The beautiful Empress Elizabeth- Sisi of Austria has been romanticized in many books and movies as a really romantic figure, but the poor lady was obsessed with beauty and her potential loss of it. In fact she was positively neurotic about it, and it is a not very well-known fact that her ladies in waiting dreaded each day when she had her long hair brushed out by them.

If the bristles showed even one hair which was on the bristle, she would go off into a weeping, wailing fit of hysteria – every day, ranging anywhere between one hour to 3 hours – excellent way to pass the time when you have nothing else constructive or sensible to do – and then she would screech at her ladies in waiting as if blaming them for her hair loss and make them stick all the fallen hair back to her scalp.

I wonder how they managed to keep sane. But then nobody had told her that there is a loss of about 100 hairs from any normal scalp, every day, especially if it is brushed. Brushing is the most harmful thing you can do to your hair, especially when you tug through tangles. That means the hairs are going to be pulled out from the roots.

However, the tradition of brushing the hair just because the aristocrats did it, and the rest of the goats had to follow the sheep was the practice followed to keep the hair dust and dirt free.

So it is time I begin to start upon my shampoo preparations. Both these utensils are not with any handles and are more like vessels with depth, but this was the way they have been made for thousands of years, and handles were a relatively addition, especially to cast-iron cooking skillets and Woks.

On the next page are 2 traditional ancient iron utensils which have been in use for generations. The larger one looks a bit wet, because I have just finished using its shampoo ingredients, which had been soaked in it overnight. These included powdered gooseberry and powdered soap nut along with an herb called Shikakai – the combination of which 3 would be enough to keep my hair growth healthy and strong, as was done traditionally.

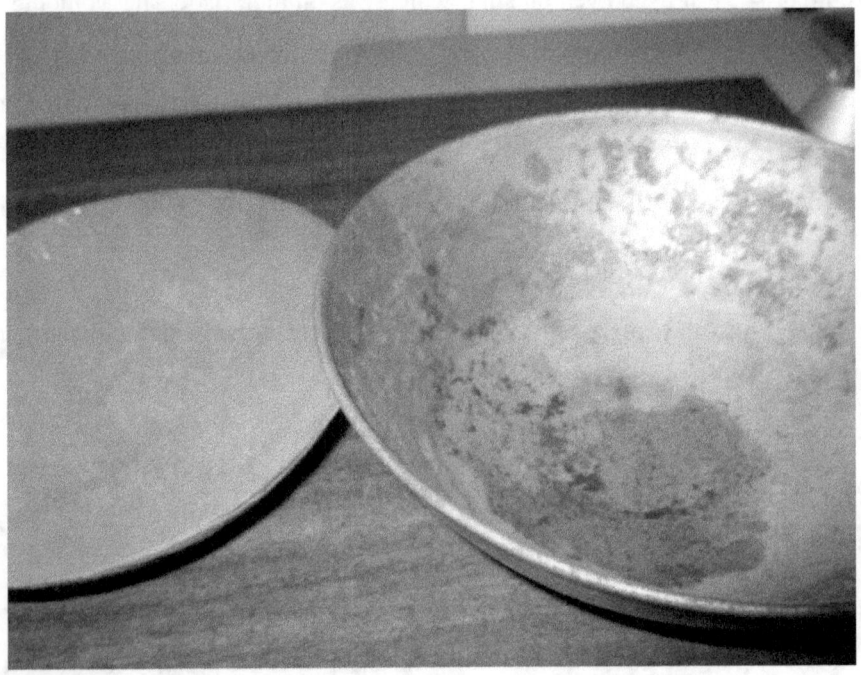

The old one on the left was found by me in one of the rooting out of ancient treasures in old village kitchens and stores. I do not know its age, but I found it in one dark, spiderweb filled dusty corner under some more really dusty and old overlooked stuff.

Someone had just put it there and forgotten it because they may have possibly bought something larger as the family expanded from the friendly neighborhood Gypsy Tinker.

The relatively large one was also garnered from one of these old ancestral homes, where it was used for ages to soak things in, this was a spare. So I requested it. When I asked my grandmother how old it was, she just shrugged her shoulders and said, well, it was in her house when she was a child, because her grandmother used to soak things in it overnight and she would not be surprised if it was even older than that.

When I was still thrilled at its nearly rust free look, she said that of course it had been made by those native Tinker Gypsy tribes through methods which are spoken, through word-of-mouth and never written down the ages. Those were the Gypsy methods used by Spanish sword makers of Toledo and once upon a time, every household in the East bought its utensils from these traditional ironworkers, Gypsy nomads, for thousands of years.

When I asked my father how they could purify iron so well that it never rusted all those millenniums ago he just said that they knew how to get rid of every bit of slag during the melting and knew the right combination of carbon, and nitrogen to put into the molten iron in order to purify it. This was not a thing which could be done in a day or even a month.

Anyway, these ancient iron utensils are not being used for cooking, but more for the soaking of traditional shampoo by me. My well seasoned traditional cast iron skillet/wok is in in the kitchen, where it belongs.

I definitely do not use any Teflon coated utensils while cooking, because I know how foolish that is, in terms of health. However much it is supposed to be touted as a convenient method of cooking, especially by our society, which is terrified of fat and oil, this chemical-based coating comes nowhere to grandma's well oiled and seasoned skillet pan made of hundred percent natural honest-to-goodness cast-iron.

In the USA, Europe, and other parts of the West, cast iron work was traditionally used for cooking in the shape of cast-iron skillets, especially in great great great and even one's own grandma's time. These were such a valuable part of the kitchen that George Washington's mother spoke about her skillet and to whom it should go in her Will.

I already spoke about the dry powdered gooseberry paste applied on the scalp and allowed to dry, before you rinsed it off to clean your hair, and keep it squeaky clean. If you are suffering from hair fall or graying, do this twice a week, for the next 3 months to get your hair follicles back to normal again and to get them growing again.

## Gooseberry Water

Just pound 25 g of dried gooseberries in a pestle and mortar. Soak them overnight in that iron utensil, of which I was talking about before. The next morning rub the gooseberries through your hands and filter the water through a thin muslin cloth.

Now you are going to rub this water slowly through your scalp, especially the root area. Allow this water to be incorporated into your scalp, for the next 10 minutes and then wash your hair with ordinary water in the summer and warm water in the winter. No shampoo, no nothing. The gooseberry water is going to do the cleaning and the nourishing.

If your hair is dry, you are going to do this once a week. If it is oily, you are going to do this twice a week. If you want, you can do this treatment, every day for a week, especially if you are looking for quick results.

But before you plan to do the shampooing, you are going to massage your hair with one hundred percent natural gooseberry oil.

# Gooseberry Oil – Natural Conditioner

You can make this in 2 ways –

# First Preparation Method – Traditional

Take a pound of green raw gooseberries, or you can grate them if you wish. Now, squeeze them through a fine muslin cloth until you have 500 g of gooseberry juice. Traditionally, this was cooked in an earthenware/clay pot, and later on in an iron pot, so use an iron pot.

Now you are going to add equal amounts of either sesame oil, olive oil, or coconut oil, or any other natural healthy oil and cook both of them together on low heat until all the watery elements in the gooseberry juice have evaporated. You will know this, when you do not hear the sound of bubbles or spluttering of water sounding from the utensil.

This means that just oil has been left and the natural goodness of gooseberries has been incorporated into the oil. Remove from heat and allow it to cool down.

Now filter this in a thin cotton muslin cloth. You are going to have greenish colored really precious oil, place in a glass bottle. Use this to condition your hair, especially before the shampoo or as a surface moisturizer.

You are going to apply it on the roots of your hair, the night before you intend to shampoo, and leave it overnight. Incidentally, when you wake up the next morning and feel your hair, it feels smooth and silky and the silky feel persists after you do the hair washing with cold or hot water and gooseberry water.

Remember that your hair should be dry, when you are applying this oil. Just rub enough warm oil in your scalp, with your fingertips so that you can have long and healthy hair, with absolutely no gray in it.

## The Second Method

Instead of fresh gooseberry juice, you are going to take a decoction of the fruit itself. For this you are going to use dried seedless gooseberries – 150 g pounded roughly in a pestle and mortar. Now you are going to put it in an iron utensil, with 600 g of water. Leave it overnight without any heating in this preliminary stage. Allow to soak for 15 hours.

The next morning, you are going to put the whole utensil along with the water and the fruit on to cook at a low heat until the water is reduced to 300 g. Now remove the utensil from the heat, and allow it to cool down.

Remember that the pulp is very useful, and should not be discarded just like that, after the cooking and boiling has been done. You are going to rub it through your fingers, and allow this mixture to filter through a muslin cloth. This is going to filter the water, and also allow the natural goodness of the fruits to be filtered along with it into the water while the pulp remains on the top of the cloth.

This is your decoction and concentrate. You are now going to put it in a glass jar and add 500 g of sesame oil, coconut oil, or any other oil of your choice like olive oil and place it on the low fire again.

Cook until all the water content is evaporated. If you want, you can add one drop of your preferred sweet smelling essential oil to this mixture.

Try this treatment of oil and shampooing – ordinary washing – every third day, and you are going to be astonished at the results, especially when your hair remains silky, healthy, shiny, bouncy, and of their natural normal color, instead of with specks of gray in them.

Also, you are going to find a positive heating and cooling effect on your eyes and head. I noticed this, but I thought it auto suggestion because I was relaxing under the head massage I was doing on my hair and scalp, and getting rid of the tension, but even when I was not tense, I found it cooling, especially in the summer.

Incidentally, I was in the mood to check up what the price of this traditional oil was online and I was astonished to see branded names – like natural herbal tonic – going for anywhere starting from $25 – up to $50 or more for 200 mg in a glass bottle.

I got hold of the dealer and told him that this was barefaced Piracy for traditionally globally beneficial oil.

"Well, he said, we are shipping these to places where they do not get gooseberries."

"Nonsense," said I, "you can get gooseberries over the world, except perhaps, maybe in desert areas."

"Well," he continued, "Maybe they do not have sesame oil or they do not have coconut oil."

I shot that down too, "They have their traditional oils, like linseed, mustard, cottonseed, sunflower, olive oil, or any other natural fruit or seed oil. If they use it for cooking, they can use it for making this hair oil."

"Ah well, they do not have the time!" "And also, they do not know the method. My family knows it. And that is why I am taking full advantage of it." He said in a triumphant voice, as if to say I have proven my point.

So now, my friends, you are going to take full advantage of the method, and you have to make the time. Don't you think your hair is worth it?

# Curing Dandruff

This is a traditional remedy, which was used extensively to cure dandruff, and still is very much en vogue. Forget about those advertisements which ask you to wash your hair and scalp with an expensive shampoo, every 7 days to get rid of dandruff.

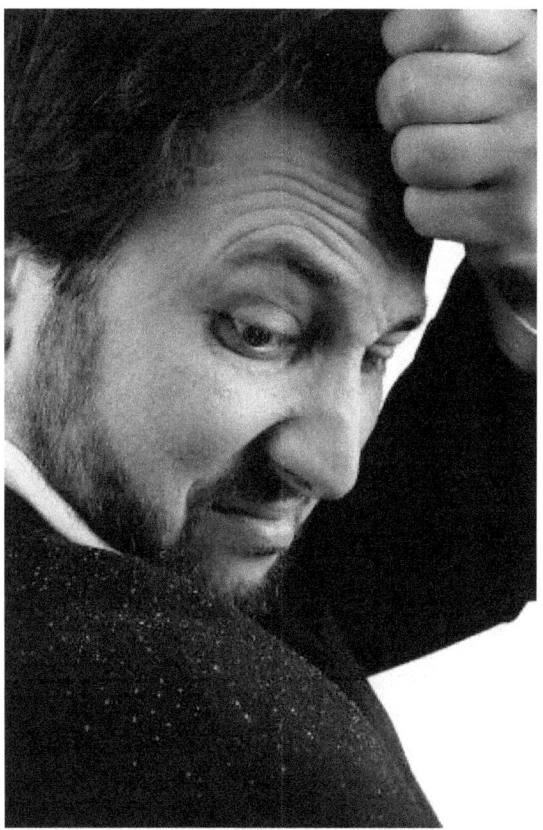

It takes 7 days for dandruff to build up. So you are shampooing it off on the seventh day, and you are so happy that your hair and scalp is dandruff free.

Take one hundred grams of your favorite oil – coconut, sesame, olive oil – and add 5 g of camphor powder to it. Mix together, and put in a glass bottle. You are going to apply just enough of this warm mixture on your scalp, for a massage twice a day, if you are suffering from a really dreadful dandruff condition.

This is first going to be done when you wash your scalp with gooseberry water, and when your hair is dry, you are going to massage the camphor oil. After that, the second massaging is going to be done when you are ready to go to sleep.

You are going to see visible improvement from the second day itself, and within the week, your scalp condition will have gone back to normal. Do this whenever you have the time, every 3 – 4 days, to prevent future dandruff buildup, when you are cured.

## Lemons

Here is another alternative – lemon juice.

Okay, let me admit it. This is one of my favorite fruit and all throughout my life, wherever I was transferred, the first thing I asked was do we have a lemon tree in our garden. Luckily we had. And in the places we did not have them, we had access to fresh lemons 24/7.

So here is the natural dandruff cure treatment alternative before you wash your hair. Ordinary lemon juice, it restores the pH balance of the skin on your scalp, while getting rid of the dandruff buildup, thanks to the acidic qualities.

You are going to take one lemon, half an hour before you shampoo – when I say shampoo, I mean washing your hair, without any soap or shampoo –

with warm water/cold water and nothing else, or alternatively gooseberry water – and rub it into your scalp, with either the lemon peel or just ordinary lemon juice.

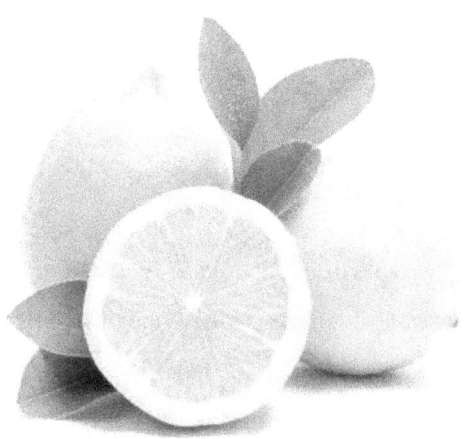

Wash your hair with warm water. Incidentally, you are going to notice that your hair will set wonderfully after you do the lemon treatment. That is why expensive spas always use lemon as the secret ingredient to set your hair, when you go there for hairstyling.

If you suffer from a chronic case of dandruff, even cooties, and dry hair, just squeeze the juice of 2 lemons in 2 L of water, and wash your hair with this, every day. One week, and your dandruff is gone, your cooties are gone, and your hair is silky and lustrous.

# Treating Lice

Here was the traditional way in which cooties were treated. Like I said before, this is the nightmare of every parent, especially when his child comes back from playing in the park/playground/school ground with all his friends and goes scratching all over the place. This cootie epidemic is going to spread all over the neighborhood, and the family.

Besides this, it is so embarrassing to just scratch an itching place and be horrified when either dandruff or cooties drop down on your shoulder, or on your book.

Take 250 g of your favorite oil – coconut, olive, sesame, mustard, linseed, and any other traditional oil – and add the juice of one lemon and a little bit of camphor to this mixture. Massage proper amounts of this mixture into your scalp every night, and in the morning, you might find dead cooties on your pillow along with flakes of dandruff, which have been loosened. You are going to wash your hair with warm water in the morning.

# Traditional Soap Nut Shampoo

Now I come to another traditional herb, known as soap nuts. Since ancient times, soap nuts have been used to clean clothes because of the soapy affect, which is gentle and mild and especially excellent to clean delicate fabrics like woollies.

Naturally, the ancients knew all about soap nut shampoo used to clean their hair and keep it squeaky clean and shiny. Also, this was an excellent dandruff, preventative.

If you suffered from hair fall, you were immediately treated to a session of soap nut shampoo, especially when you suffered from lots of hair fall. This treatment was done every 4 days until you found your fallen-out-during-the-night hair not lying there crying on your pillow when you woke up every morning.

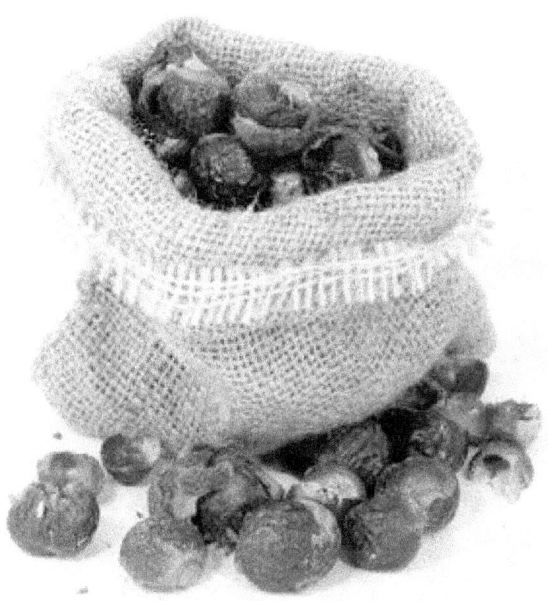

**Soap Nuts**

To make the soap nut shampoo, you are going to use the skin of the soap nut broken up into small pieces, soaked overnight in the proportion of one part soap nut skin, one part water. Soaking it in an iron utensil is excellent, especially when you are soaking 2 parts of gooseberry powder in this mixture at the same time. The third is shikakai, 3 parts shikakai which is a traditional herb now available globally under this name, but even if you do not have this last, no worry.

In the morning, you are going to rub the soap nut pulp and gooseberry powder well, if you want, or you may want to heat it a bit, so that you get an even more powerful concentrate, so much better.

This is how you are going to wash your hair with this water. You are going to take half of this portion and rub your hair for 5 – 10 minutes to get rid of all the grime, dust, and oil. Then wash it with ordinary water. Repeat with the rest of the shampoo to make it totally grime free and squeaky clean.

Then give your hair a last rinse with a water shower. Do this twice every week for long and grimy hair, every second or third day, for better hair growth and whenever else you wish.

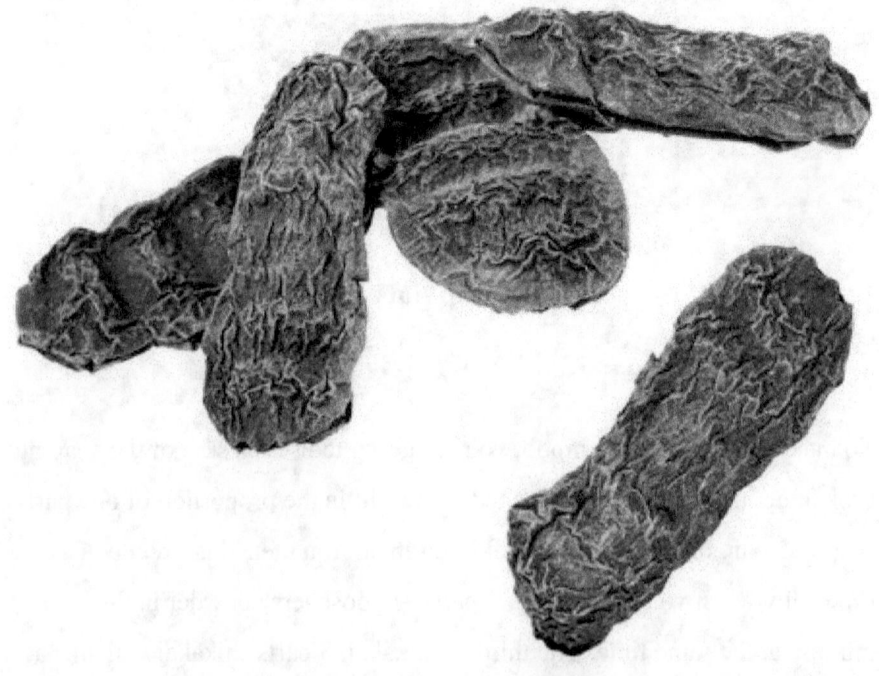

**Acacia concinna- Shikakai**

If you do not want to use soap nut, you can use a combination of Shikakai powder and powdered gooseberry – 25 g of each – pound a little bit together in a pestle and mortar, and soak them overnight in 500 g of water. You are going to filter this mixture the next morning and rub the water all over your scalp and hair. Wash your hair after 20 minutes. After that, you may want to apply your favorite gooseberry oil – the one we made from the formula given above, to your hair, and have really nice silky, well conditioned and tangle free hair.

But, you say, when you apply hair to your scalp, it is absolutely sticky, and you do not like the feeling. No problem. After you have washed your hair, just dip your fingers in the warm oil. Rub it on to your skull and the surface of your hair when it is still wet. Do a little bit of massage, especially over the surface.

After that, stand under the shower with your comb and get rid of all the tangles, with your hair still wet. Be careful, because this is the time when your hair are going to fall, but do not worry, because unless you have chunks full of hair coming out straight from the roots, as it happens during chemotherapy, you do not have to worry.

Your hair is now smooth and tangle free, and well conditioned. Best of all, they have plenty of nourishing material on which to feed. They are also squeaky clean. You are going to be really pleased with the hair growth of your hair from now on.

This is excellent in the summers. I am starting this right now, even though it is still winter so that by the time it is time for vacations in the summer heat, – for 4 months – I am going to have really healthy, shiny, long, and manageable hair without any sort of gray.

Along with this, here is the supporting diet, which is going to help your hair grow. Eat a radish with pepper and salt every day. It is going to take 3 – 4 months, if your hair is not very healthy in the first place. This is the amount of time it is going to take for your hair follicles to start growing again with this natural nourishment and treatment. The best thing about eating the radishes is that you are going to find your state of hunger improved and you are not going to suffer from flatulence or constipation.

Eat radishes only if they suit you.

## Yogurt Shampoo – Natural Hair Darkener

Lots of milk products in your diet are excellent for your hair and skin.

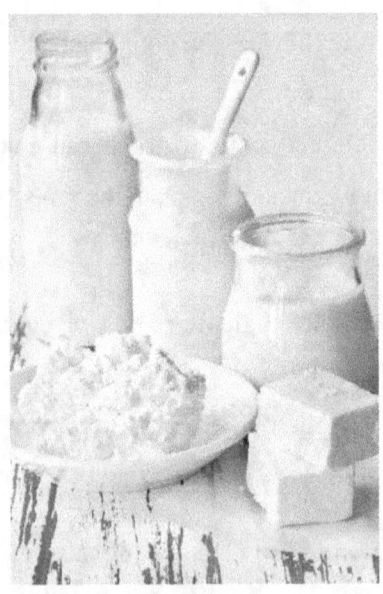

Here is another alternative with which you can clean your hair and has been in use for thousands of years. Just ordinary yogurt.

You are going to take one hundred grams of yogurt and put 3 ground peppercorns in it. Wash your hair with this mixture, and then after that, wash your hair again with warm water, once a week. I remember my grandmother doing this to her hair, every Sunday and we just loved to touch her smooth and silky hair. Absolutely no tangles, and black still in it, even though she was in her eighties. This is a natural hair darkener . But then she was not using gooseberry or any hair darkening agent in our neck of the woods – 200 miles away from civilization in the middle of the darkest, deepest forests, 4000 feet above sea level.

So she was using her traditional "soap" for hair cleanliness and conditioning.

## Pepper and Salt Hair

If you are suffering from pepper and salt hair, you are going to take the juice of 2 lemons and add 2 cups of hot water to the mixture. Now wet your hair thoroughly and use this mixture as a shampoo all over your scalp and hair.

**Do not wash your hair, with warm/cold water as the last rinse like you did in the previous remedies. Just dry it with your towel.**

Now comb your hair slowly, drying your hair in the shade. Do not use a hairdryer, because seriously, this is the best way in which you can dehydrate your hair and scalp, and expose the follicles to direct heat, thus killing them effectively. We are so used to blow drying our hair that we forget that our hair hates the trauma of heat applied to it in any sort, including dry air from a blow dryer or a hairdryer. As that is what makes the beauty and salon industry rub its hands in glee. They are going to dye your hair, condition your hair, sell you hair restorers and hair conditioners and all that advertising jazz,just because you used a blow dryer.

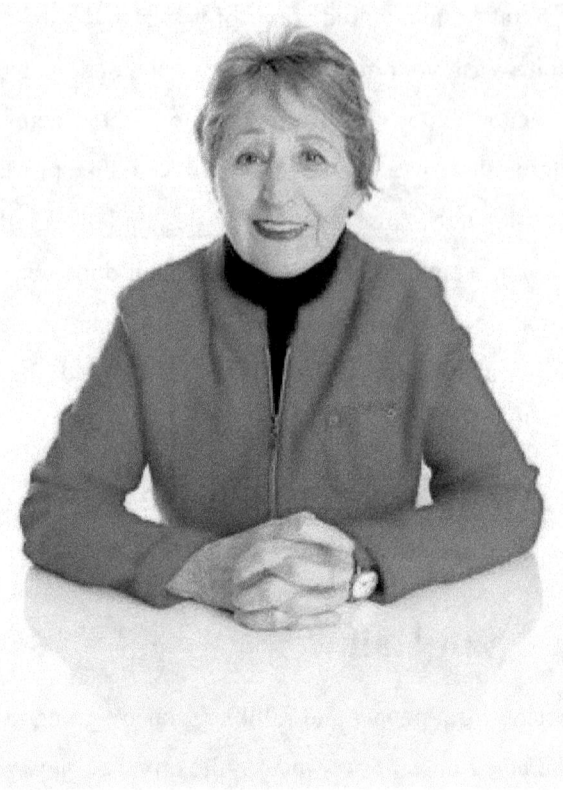

Instead, do some gentle wiping on your hair with a soft towel. Dry it in the shade, while combing it gently. Enjoy the silky feel. Do this twice a week and you are soon going to find your hair, regaining its natural color.

## Lemon Oil Supporting Treatment

Along with this, you are going to do these supporting treatments – take some lemon peels, and dip them in your favorite hair oil and put them in the shade for the next 10 days. Then filter it, and use this oil – lemon oil on your scalp to darken your hair follicles and get rid of all the white.

Traditionally, this oil could be used, and premature graying was stopped permanently with another oil treatment.

For this you would take 300 g of coconut oil or your favorite oil. To this, you would add 1 tablespoon of roughly ground pepper. You would heat this oil so that you could get the pepper extract into the coconut.

Filter after it has been boiled once and cooled down. Apply this, on your scalp with your fingertips, before you go to sleep and you are going to grow old in years, but never visibly as seen through your hair.

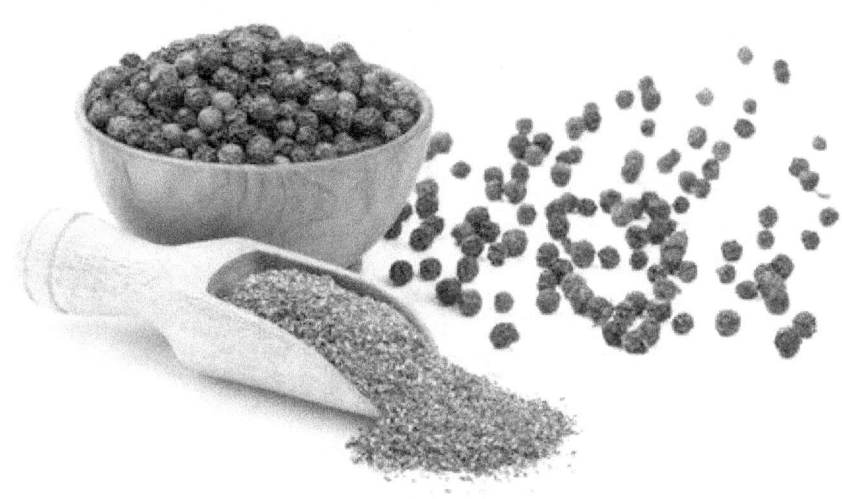

**You never knew that pepper was an excellent spice for encouraging hair growth, did you?**

# Final Rinse

There are plenty of natural products, which have been used traditionally as a final rinse, including beer, lemon water, and even Apple cider vinegar. These are all traditional and well-known. So what you are going to do is take the juice of one lemon with a couple of drops of vinegar, in a glass of warm water in the winters and cold water in the summers and use this as the final rinse, after your hair is clean. Then give it the absolutely last shower to get rid of any vestiges of grime and oil and any other extras, before you begin toweling.

This is excellent to cure dandruff and also the best thing is that you are going to find your hair getting less grimy than usual.

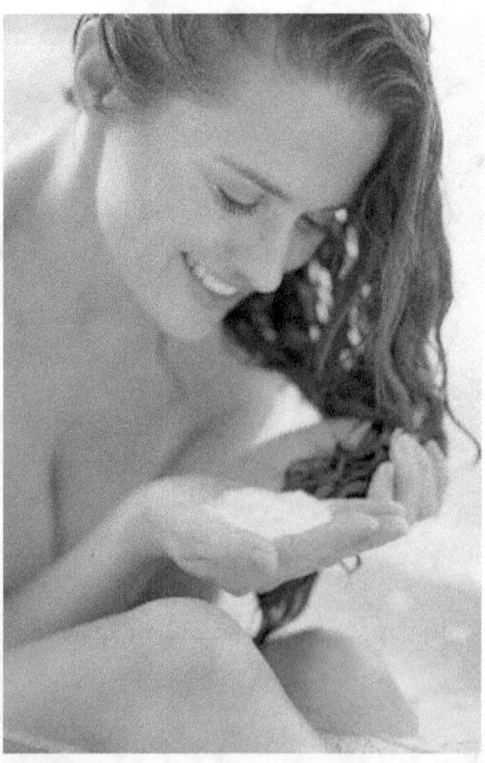

# Fullers Earth Shampoo

Using a paste of fuller's earth to wash your hair has been en vogue for centuries. For this you are going to take one hundred grams of Fuller's Earth. This is a natural earth which has been traditionally used by sheep herders'- fullers- traditionally to clean the dirt and grime from shorn sheep's wool, or to get rid of all the oil in any job, which includes a mixture of oil, dust, and grime.

In ancient times, this earth was used extensively as a shampoo, because of its slick feel, to clean the hair of grime, and also to give the hair a softer shine.

So use one hundred grams of traditional earth – it is creamy/yellow in color. If you find blocks of this earth with streaks of brown, do not buy it. Those are the impurities – is going to be soaked in a bowl full of water. In 2 hours it is going to swell up and the pieces of earth are going to break up into a powdery pulp.

Use your fingers to rub it into a smooth paste without any lumps. The paste should be thick enough to spread all over your hair and rub the surface slowly so that the oil and grime is cleaned away. Do this for 5 minutes. Then wash your hair with warm water in the winter and cold water in the summer.

If your hair is really not clean in the first rubbing, do that again. The second rubbing is going to be totally effective. Traditionally, this was the way in which the ancients washed their hair twice a week and kept the shine. You are going to be surprised to see the effect on your head, hair, and even condition of hair seen visibly in the first wash itself.

# Chickpea – Gram Flour Shampoo

This is the traditional way in which hair are washed in areas where you have plenty of chickpeas, especially the Middle East, where this is an important ingredient of hummus and other traditional chickpea based dishes.

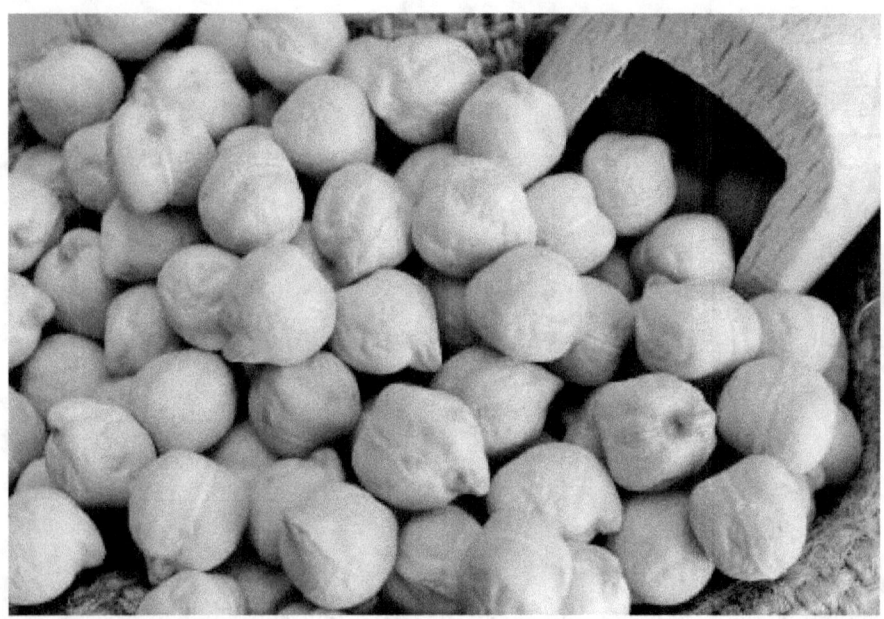

For this, chickpea flour is used. Chickpea flour has been in use since ancient times as the base for cleaning the skin as a paste where it was mixed with milk, cream, lemon, and salt, and rubbed all over the surface of the skin to get rid of the dead skin, dirt, and grime.

If this can be done on your skin, it can be done on your hair too. You are going to be using chickpea flour, twice a week. Apply a thick paste of this flour made up in water, on your hair and scalp. Allow to rest for one hour, and then wash your hair with warm/cold water. This means that you are going to have clean, healthy, and dark hair as well as get rid of any sort of scalp problems, including infections on the scalp.

# Baldness

If baldness is genetic, and you find yourself balding in your twenties and thirties, here is a traditional remedy, which you may want to try out, if you can get a little bit of opium, which has been in use as a traditional medicine for millenniums.

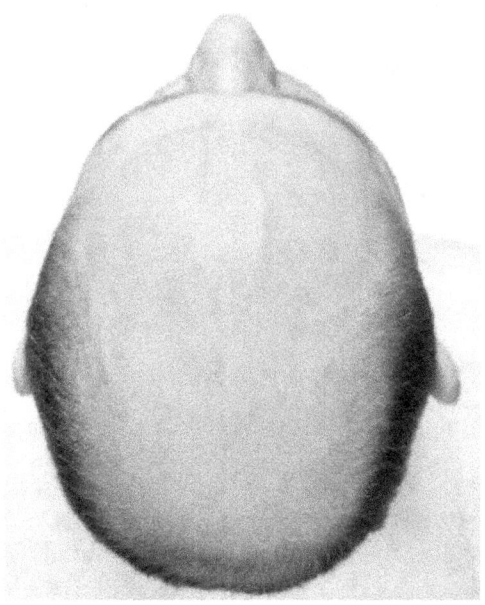

Incidentally, the usage of opium as a recreational drug started by the British in the late eighteenth century to get the Chinese addicted, so that they could continue business in a land which did not welcome foreigners, especially those from the West. Two million Chinese were addicted to opium within 3 years. In fact, we can blame these traders for the future drug addicts, forever more, who began to use medicinal drugs as recreational drugs.

And then they still shriek about the totally unfair Boxer Revolution in the early twentieth century, where the Chinese decided to throw these ruthless and greedy traders out of China, and cry – what have we done to deserve this, how could those Chinese treat us like that, we just came as simple traders, trading in tea and feeding them opium instead.

Anyway, if the baldness is due to skin infections, or any other health cause, try adding a little bit of opium to lemon juice and apply it all over the balding areas to encourage the growth of hair follicles.

## Traditional Natural Hair Dye

Chemical hair dyes which you get in the market are capable of creating skin problems. Some of these constituents may also cause allergies especially in sensitive skin.

I found this recipe in a 600 year old Persian medicine book, made by traditional medicine men, where this dye was called *Khi'ja'ab*. And here I was, thinking that the traditional dye was henna leaves to give dark and white hair a red tint.

Anyway, all of us know that henna is the traditional tinting natural conditioner turning your head russet instead of gray. This traditional hair dye is again made of gooseberries.

Take about 500 g of raw/dried gooseberries, and soak them overnight. The next morning, you are going to rub the pulp with your fingers and wash your hair with this mixture. Do this twice a week until your hair starts to grow darker. Along with this, you are going to eat one raw gooseberry everyday or drink one spoonful of gooseberry powder in a glass full of water.

To make the dye you are going to take one kilo of gooseberry juice, to which you are going to add 1 kg of clarified butter. This clarified butter is just pure concentrated butter fat heated to a golden yellow color. Now remember, this is a very powerful concentrate. To this mixture, you are going to add 250 g of licorice powder.

Heat them slowly on low heat until all the water dries. Filter and put in a glass bottle. This is the best dye which you are going to apply all over your skull/scalp, like you would do any other dye to color your hair. Your hair does not appear dark, but they will start darkening within a number of days. Also, apart from premature gain, your hair is going to start going dark from the roots and follicles.

# Henna Dye

Henna has been in use for millenniums in order to decorate the hands and feet. It is also called mehendi, all over the world. Naturally, this is the best hair natural dyer, conditioner, and tinting agent.

If you want another traditional dye, you are going to use a mixture of powdered gooseberry, some leaves of henna and some leaves of the neem tree. You are going to mix them along with milk. Apply this paste all over the area, where you want the hair to grow dark again. Wash this with warm water after the paste has dried within an hour.

Do this twice a week and you are going to find your hair growing dark again within 2 months.

Also, instead, you can try dough made out of water and dried henna powder and dried gooseberry. Knead it into dough, instead of making it into a wet paste. Apply it all over with a little bit more water on your scalp and allow to dry for the next 4 months.

Now wash it with ordinary water. After that, you are going to apply gooseberry oil on your hair. Do this just once a week, and you are going to find your hair color changing slowly and steadily to dark instead of white.

# Conclusion

This book has given you plenty of interesting knowledge on traditional haircare and scalp care methods.

I have not spoken much about diet here, but in ancient times, the people ate green leafy vegetables, eggs, milk products, and high-protein diets in order to keep themselves healthy. So look for natural and organic foods, especially milk, eggs, and organic meat to keep your system healthy.

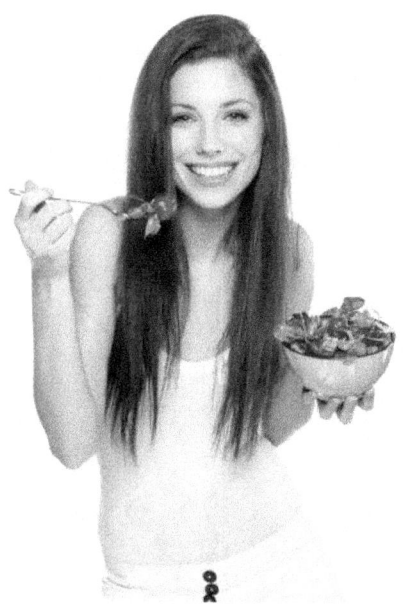

If you starve yourself, especially in that stupid bid to be a size 0, in order to look as skeletal as a famine survivor – I cannot imagine people doing this on purpose, when they have food around them and in nature and your body needs and demands natural vitamins, fats, carbohydrates, minerals, and nutrients in order to survive, – the first effect is going to show up on your skin and after that upon your hair.

So it is of no use buying vitamin supplements, and expensive hair conditioners and other hair repair items to keep your hair healthy, when the rest of your body is starving of nutrients. Get sensible, start eating healthy, and do not neglect your health, just because society or some silly idea of fashion en vogue demands it.

Live Long and Prosper!

# Author Bio

**Dueep Jyot Singh**  is a Management and IT Professional who managed to gather Postgraduate qualifications in Management and English and Degrees in Science, French and Education while pursuing different enjoyable  career options like being an hospital administrator,  IT,SEO and HRD  Database Manager/ trainer, movie , radio and TV scriptwriter, theatre  artiste and public speaker, lecturer in French, Marketing and Advertising, ex-Editor of Hearts On Fire (now known as Solstice) Books Missouri USA, advice columnist and cartoonist, publisher and Aviation School trainer, ex-moderator on Medico.in, banker, student  councilor ,travelogue writer … among other things!

One fine morning, she decided that she had enough of killing herself by Degrees and went back to her first love—writing. It's more enjoyable! She already has 48 published academic and 14 fiction- in- different- genre books under her belt.

When she is not designing websites or making Graphic design illustrations for clients , she is browsing through old bookshops hunting for treasures, of which she has an enviable collection – including R.L. Stevenson, O.Henry, Dornford Yates, Maurice Walsh, De Maupassant, Victor Hugo, Sapper, C.N. Williamson,  "Bartimeus" and the crown of her collection- Dickens "The Old Curiosity Shop," and "Martin Chuzzlewit" and so on… Just call her "Renaissance Woman"  - collecting herbal remedies, acting like Universal Helping Hand/Agony Aunt, or escaping to her dear mountains for a bit of exploring, collecting herbs and plants, and trekking.

# Check out some of the other JD-Biz Publishing books

Gardening Series on Amazon

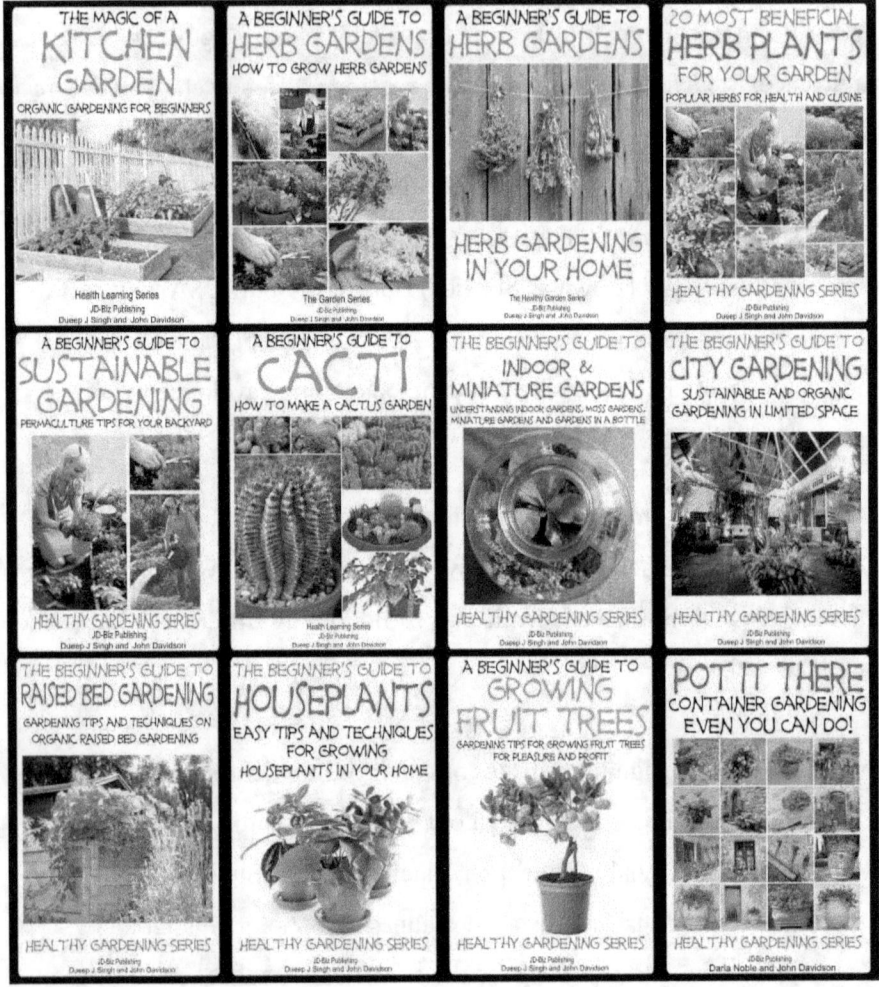

## Download Free Books!

## http://MendonCottageBooks.com

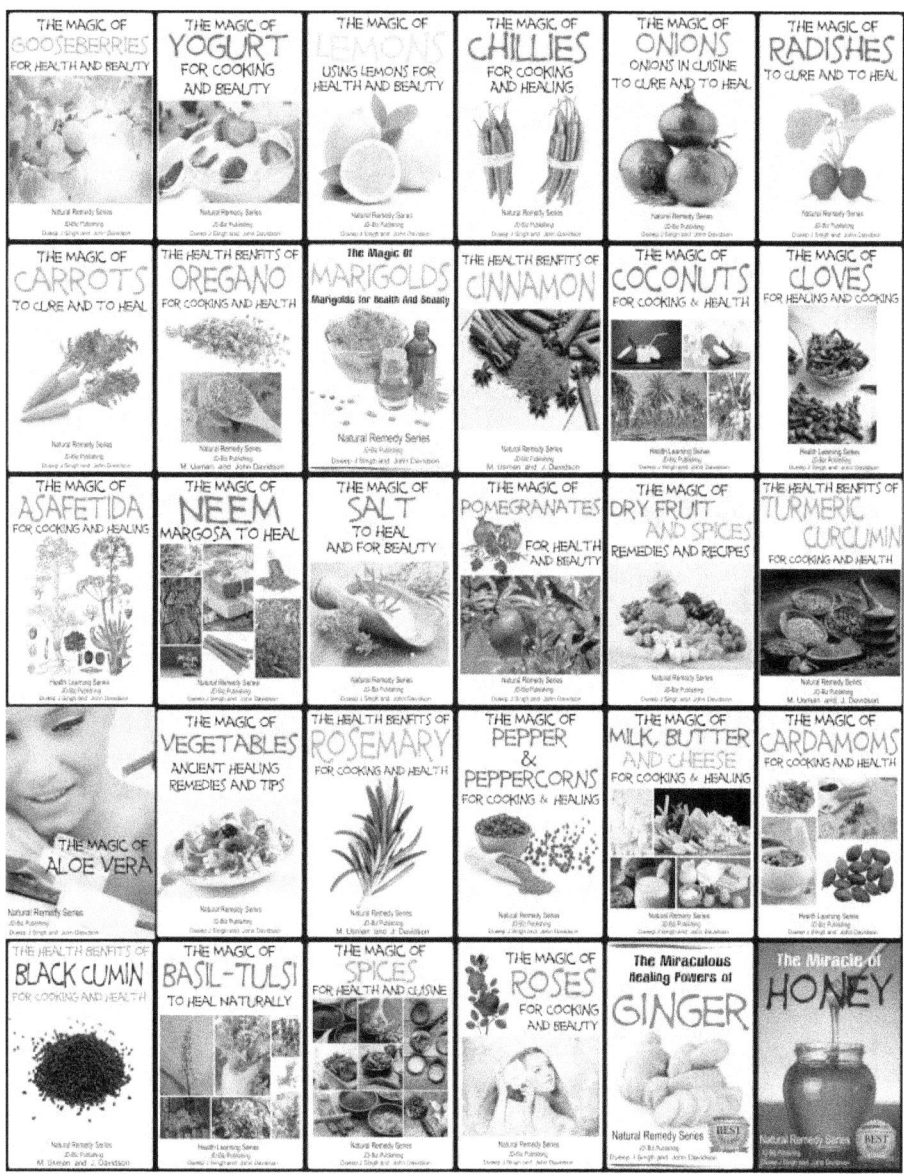

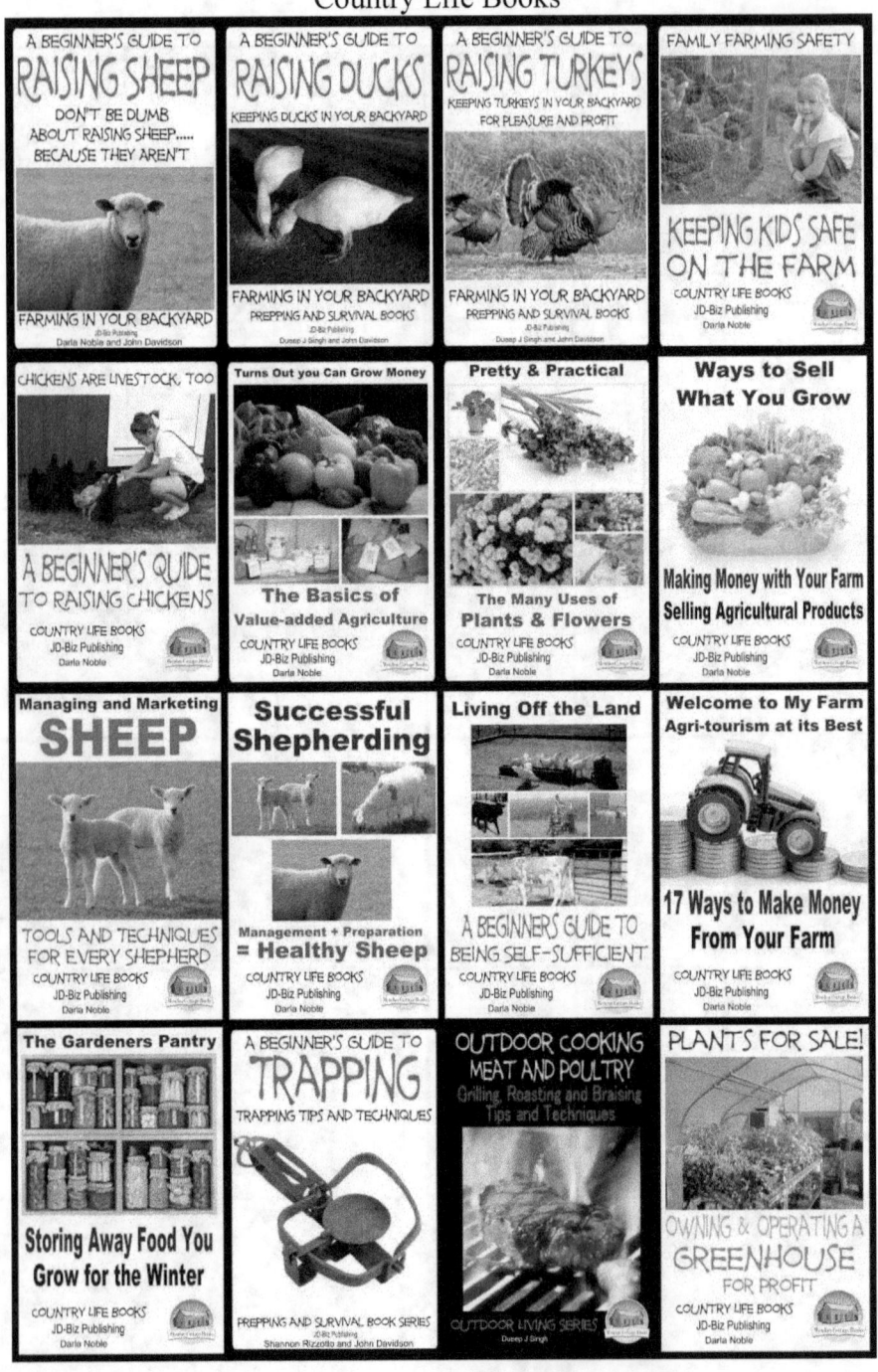

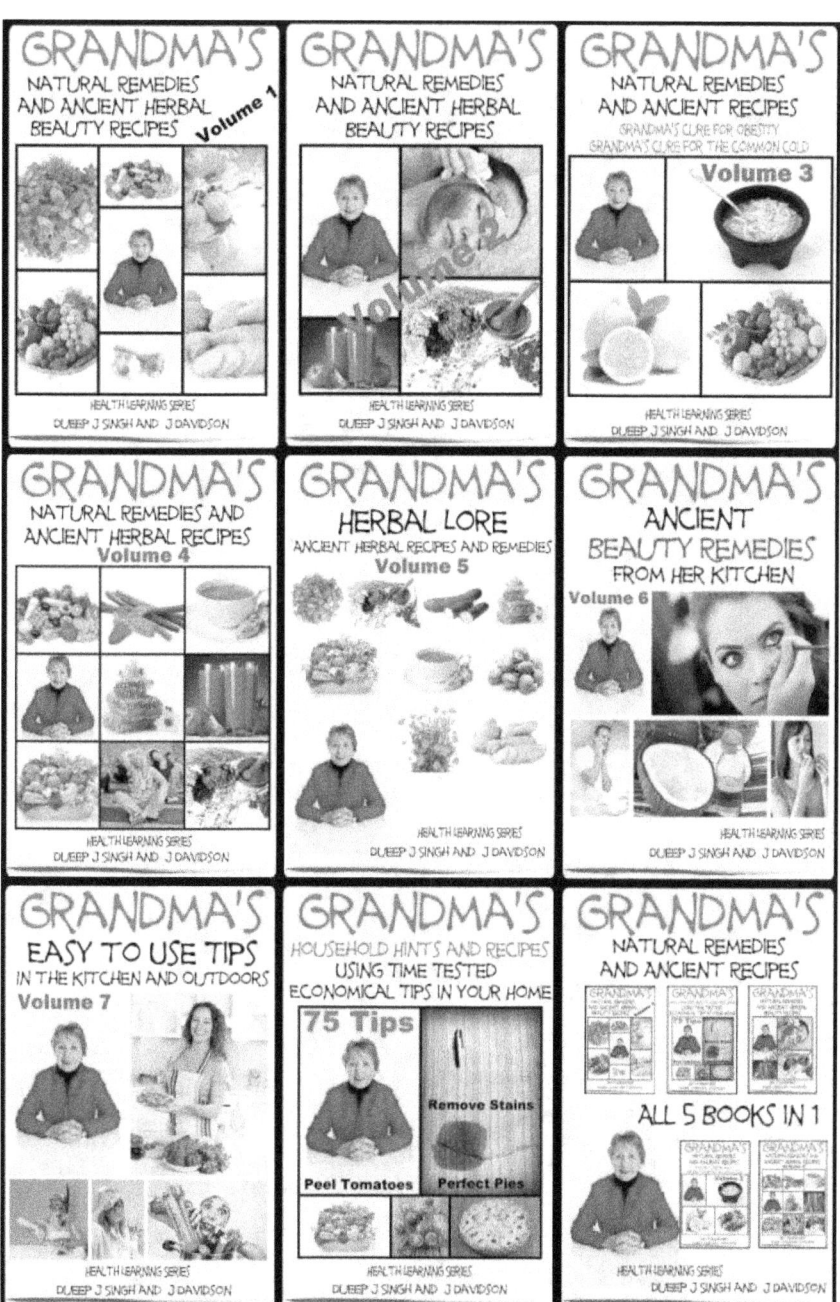

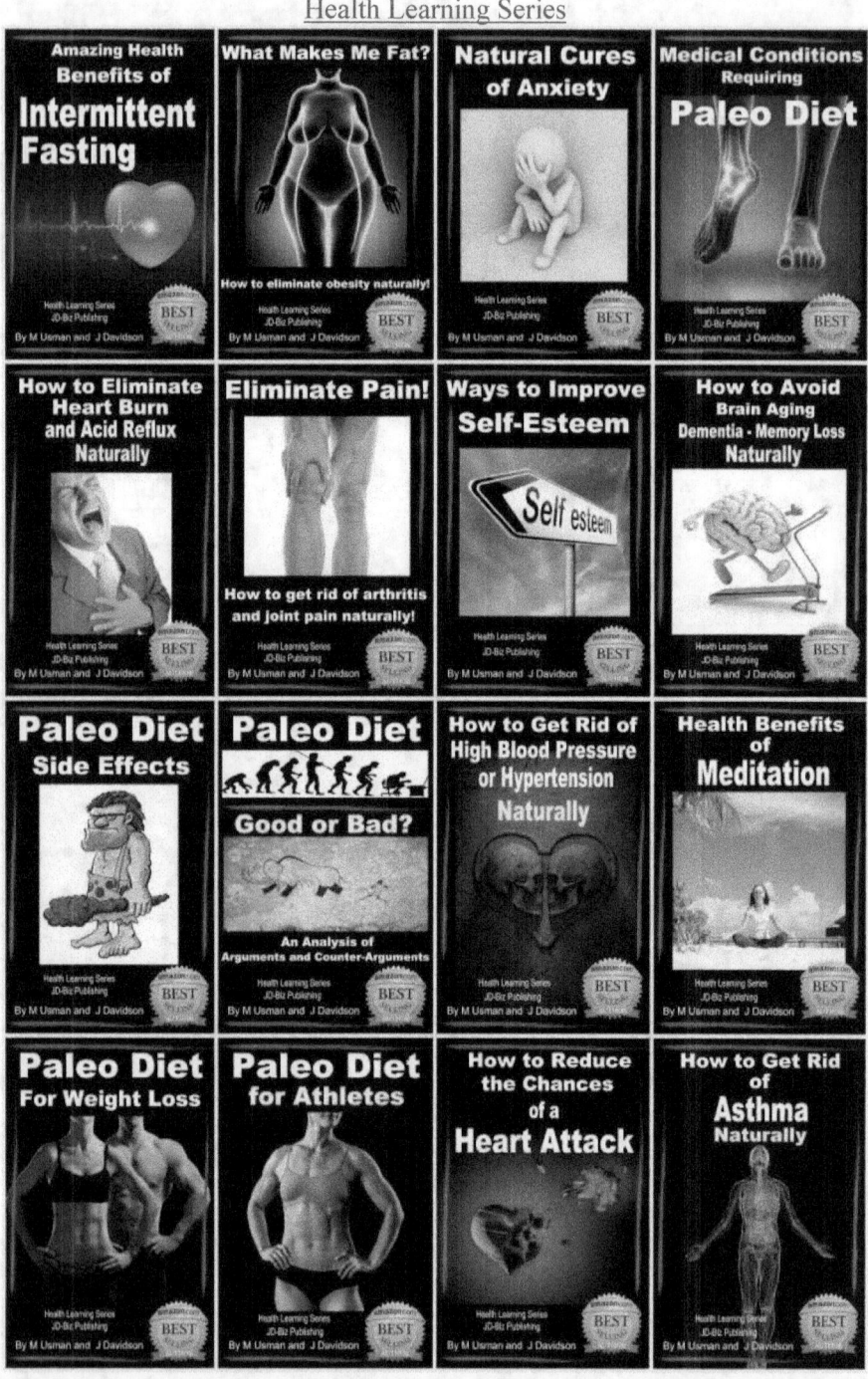

# Amazing Animal Book Series

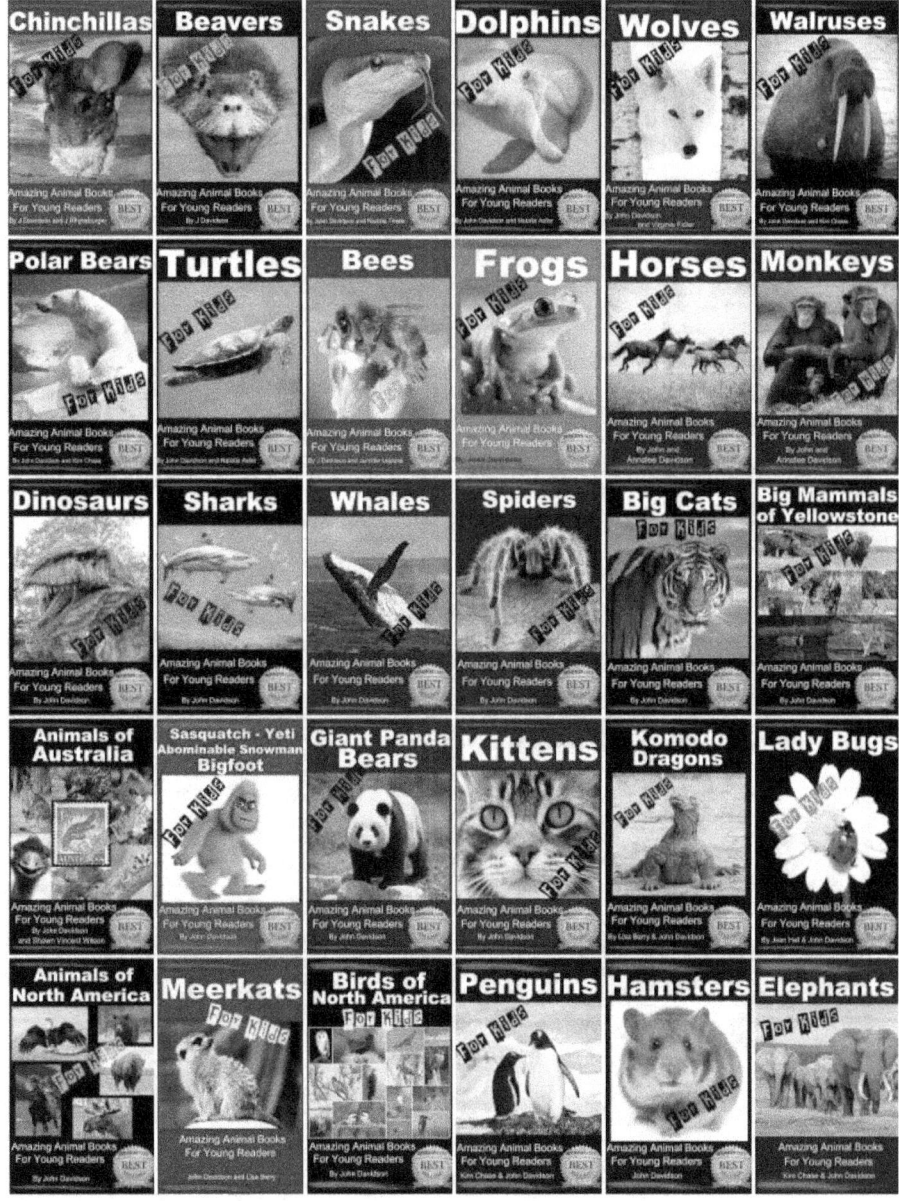

# Learn To Draw Series

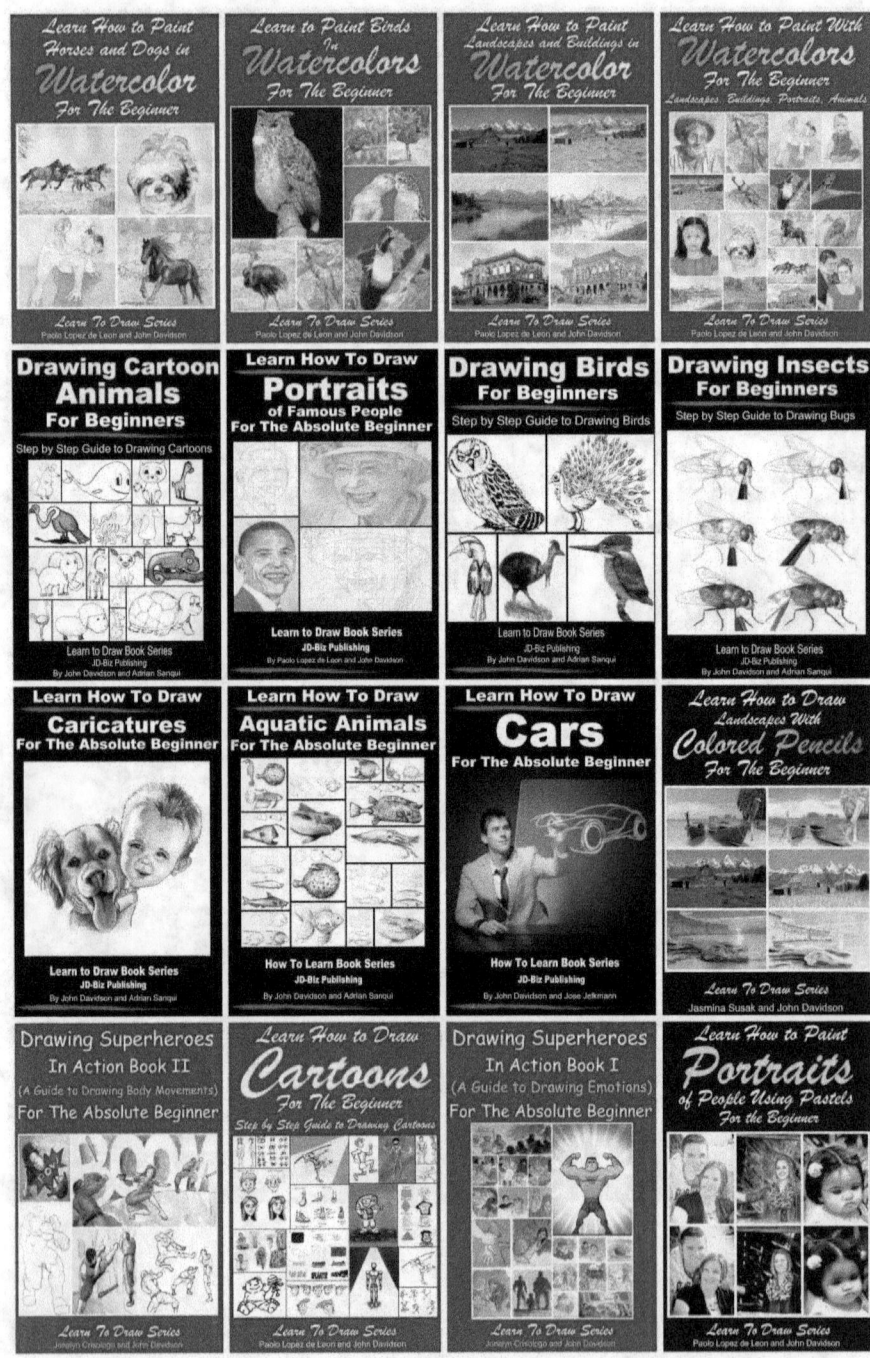

# How to Build and Plan Books

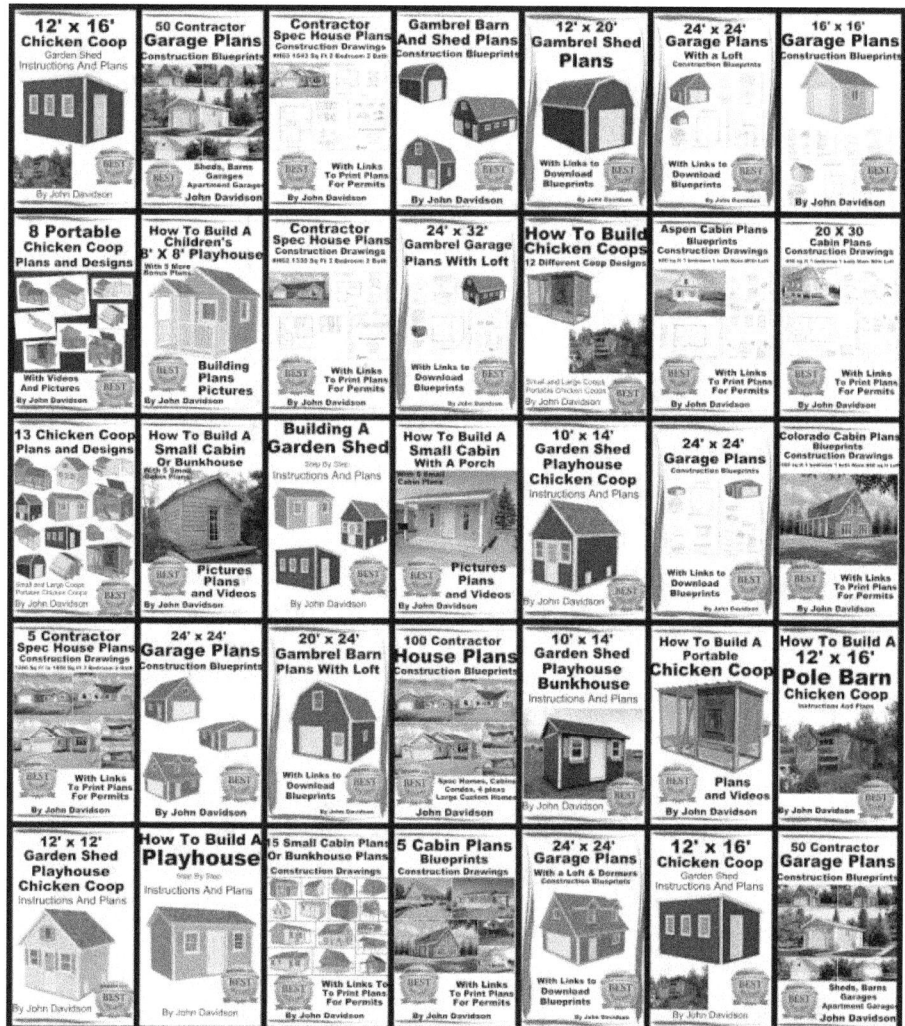

# Entrepreneur Book Series

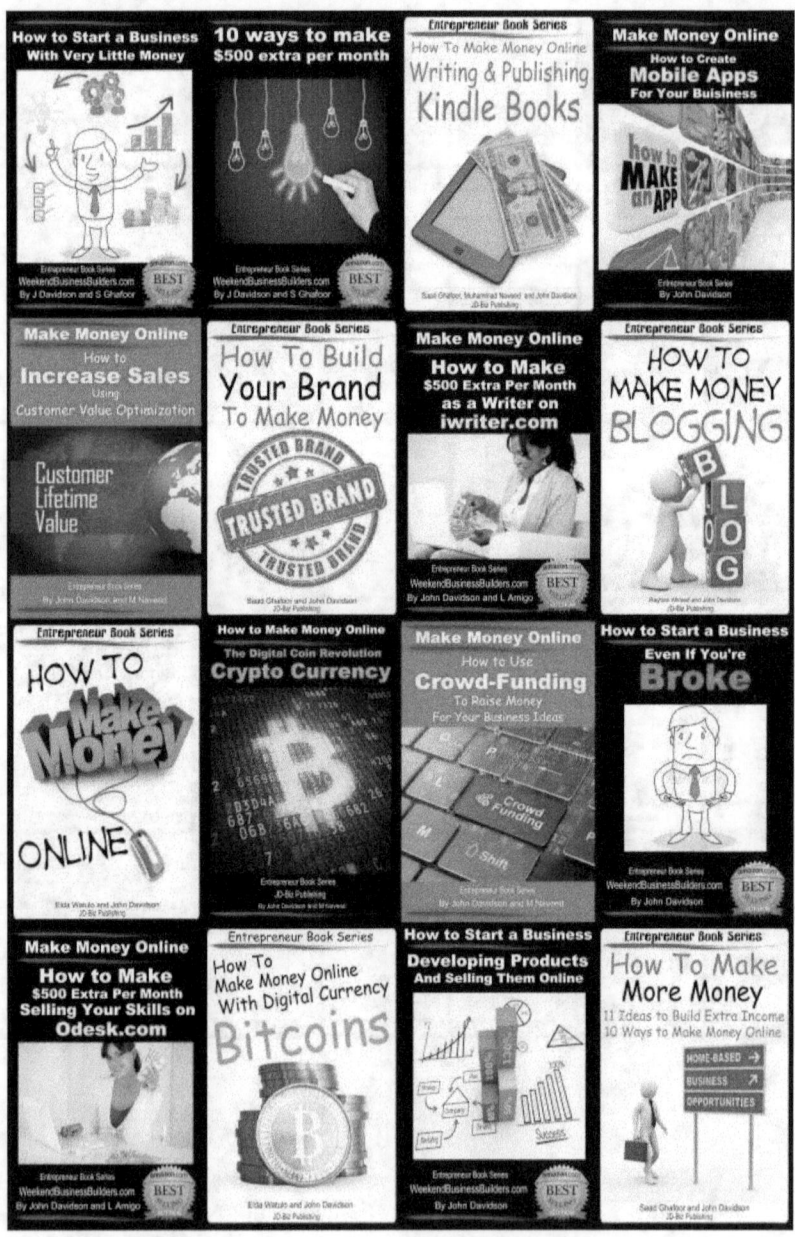

**Our books are available at**

1. Amazon.com

2. Barnes and Noble

3. Itunes

4. Kobo

5. Smashwords

6. Google Play Books


# Download Free Books!

# http://MendonCottageBooks.com

# Publisher

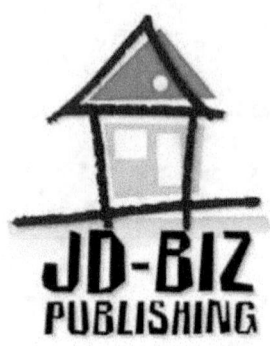

JD-Biz Corp

P O Box 374

Mendon, Utah 84325

http://www.jd-biz.com/

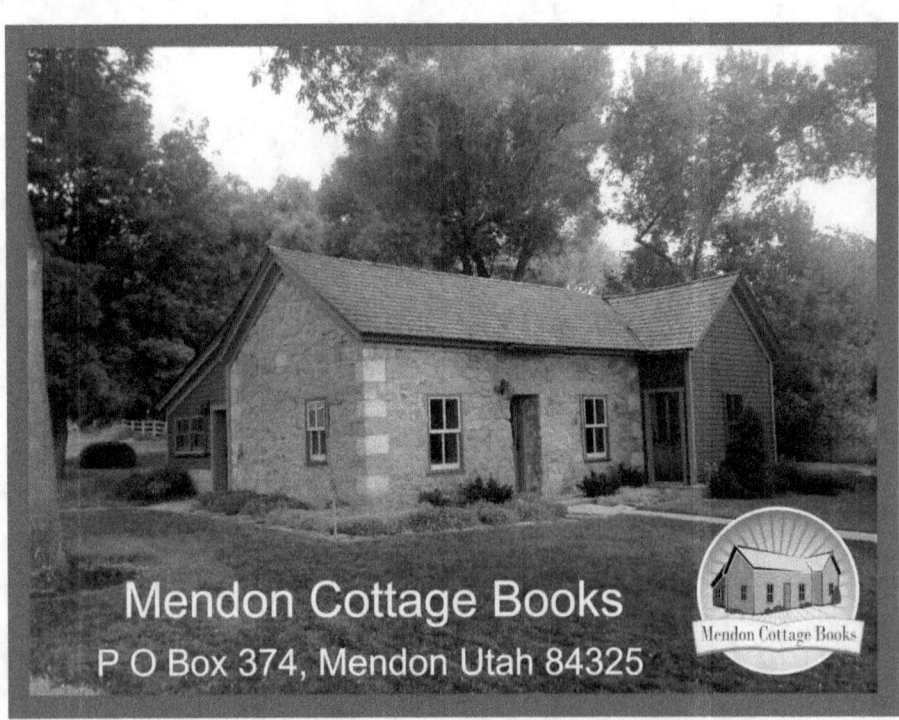

Mendon Cottage Books

P O Box 374, Mendon Utah 84325

www.ingramcontent.com/pod-product-compliance
Lightning Source LLC
Chambersburg PA
CBHW071249280526
45788CB00004B/1650